Nicolae Popescu
Grigore-Alexandru Popescu

Consonantist Psychosomatics

AF168230

Nicolae Popescu
Grigore-Alexandru Popescu

Consonantist Psychosomatics

Contribution of doctor Stefan Odobleja to the concept of psychosomatics

LAP LAMBERT Academic Publishing

Impressum / Imprint

Bibliografische Information der Deutschen Nationalbibliothek: Die Deutsche Nationalbibliothek verzeichnet diese Publikation in der Deutschen Nationalbibliografie; detaillierte bibliografische Daten sind im Internet über http://dnb.d-nb.de abrufbar.

Bibliographic information published by the Deutsche Nationalbibliothek: The Deutsche Nationalbibliothek lists this publication in the Deutsche Nationalbibliografie; detailed bibliographic data are available in the Internet at http://dnb.d-nb.de.

Coverbild / Cover image: www.ingimage.com

Verlag / Publisher:
LAP LAMBERT Academic Publishing
ist ein Imprint der / is a trademark of
OmniScriptum GmbH & Co. KG
Heinrich-Böcking-Str. 6-8, 66121 Saarbrücken, Deutschland / Germany
Email: info@lap-publishing.com

Herstellung: siehe letzte Seite /
Printed at: see last page
ISBN: 978-3-659-75488-3

NICOLAE POPESCU   GRIGORE-ALEXANDRU POPESCU

CONSONANTIST PSYCHOSOMATICS
Contribution of doctor Stefan Odobleja to the concept of psychosomatics

Translation: Dana BREHAR – CIOFLEC, MD, PhD
Technical editore: engineer Cornelia CIUCIU
Cover I.   engineer Cornelia CIUCIU; Psychosomatic interactions. Source: adaptated
after Şt. Odobleja (1982): Psihologia consonantistă, Ed. Ştiinţifică şi Enciclopedică,
Bucureşti, p. 425.

Correspondence to:
Nicolae Popescu
consultant in Family Medicine, doctor in medical science, Individual
Medical Practice DR POPESCU NICOLAE
Address: Bdl. Carol I, 61, Drobeta Turnu-Severin, Mehedinţi
Phone: +4 0722213910
E-mail address: npopescu_mf_kt@yahoo.com

2

CONTENTS

1. FOREWORD

My interest for Stefan Odobleja and his work has started since I was at highschool, when I was a colleague of the future engineer Radu Caltea, whose father was a dermatologist and lived next door to dr.Stefan Odobleja with whom he had long discussions on the works of the scientist. In 1968, in my colleague's house, I saw the two volumes of „Psychologie consonantiste", originally printed in French in Lugoj, by personal contribution and distributed by „Libraire Maloine" in Paris between 1938-1939 which had been received by the father of my colleague, dr. Constantin Caltea from his neighbour, dr. Stefan Odobleja, in 72, Decebal Street, today renamed as Stefan Odobleja Street.

It was a chance for me when I went to the same highschool with the great scientist i.e. „Traian" National College in Drobeta Turnu Severin, but this happened after 50 years, and then I followed the same faculty, the Faculty of Medicine and Pharmacy Bucharest, the Army Medical Institute. Thus, I followed a military career, as Stefan Odobleja did, except that his career as a military physician also included a period during the second World War, both on the Eastern and on the Western front, after Romania changed sides, and my career as an army physician only occurred in times of peace.

In 1981, while I was attending a course, I found that in the museum dedicated to great personalities of Romanian military medicine, there was a well desearved place for the one who had the first generalised cybernetic vision and elaborated the first cybernetic psychology and to this place I brought my contribution with photos of moments from his life and activity.

During the period 1999-2006 I led a research at the Customs Police where I was working at that time as a military physician, inspired by Stefan Odobleja's work and under the guidance of the late Prof. Mircea Ancusa.

A human being, throughout his evolution, was and still is undergoing a continuous process of adaptation to environmental (geographical, climate-related, social) changes which may act as trigger agents, process which has been defined by Hans Selye as the,, general adaptation syndrome", and by Stefan Odobleja in „Psychologie consonantiste", the terms consonance-dissonance signifying health balance.

My reasons for choosing to entitle my PhD thesis „**Occupational Stress Factors and the Possible Occurence of Psychosomatic and Behavioural Pathology in**

Customs Police Staff Members" may be grouped in four categories linked to *profession, military activity, transition* from centralised economy to democracy and *free market economy*, as well as the psychsomatic category as preferential approach for patients from the perspective of indepth studies in this field.

A. The first is the main occupation, namely family medicine, preceded by my activity as general practitioner in various army structures. The family physician (FP) grants patients access to healthcare, as the first specialist coming into contact with the patient and thus ensuring a great part of the current healthcare services. Unlike specialists in various fields, the FP analyses the patient as a whole thus having the possibility to discover connections between phenomena, such as those between psychological and somatic factors in psychosomatic diseases. Moreover, the FP ensures healthcare continuity and has the possibility to know positive and negative aspects confronting the healthy or diseased individual within his family and society, throughout a long period, sometimes from birth until death. To sum up, the FP is „the physician of the family, all problems included".

In this context, he can widely and truly promote the principles of psychosomatic medicine as „there is no other veritable general medicine than psychosomatic medicine" and „psychosomatic medicine as a whole is the most elaborate form of general medicine".

B. The second motivation is based on the activity within the army which started during my student years at the Medical Military Institute of the University of Medicine and Pharmacy Bucharest (1970-1976) where I met the rigour of a military institution of higher education and went through the specific adaptation phases of life in the army.

After graduation, I was enrolled in an elite department of the National Defense Ministry, i.e. „frontier troops" where I started my career as a military physician (1976-1983). Together with daily healthcare, promoting and maintaining the health status of the assisted troops was of utmost importance; for this, the risk factors of diseases, primarily the psychological structure of the military staff had to be known because the main task was guarding the frontiers for which soldiers were given arms with war ammunition. Thus, if physical and mental health status were unknown, the premises for unwanted events could be created (desertion, or other deviations, minor or severe injuries during manipulation of arms, homicides, suicides, etc.). Based upon the periodic morbidity study I was able to assess that there was a correlation between risk factors and the recorded morbidity.

For several years (1983-1989), I was active as teritorial military staff (CMJ), where the main activity was the selection and occupational counselling of young recruits upon enrolment and of young people selected for teaching institutions of the army.

Among the specific techniques and methods used for selection, psychological tests had an important role in the detection of personality disorders, premorbid personalities, or for deciding the required abilities for repartition in military units. Of course, these tests preceded a complex medical evaluation and those with various problems detected during testing were subjected to a well conducted interview in the psychiatric office. The tests applied included personality tests, mental level and stability, integration and dynamics assessment.

Another important period I went through in military institutions was that during which I coordinated medical services in a large frontier unit (1989-2000). Together with specific emergency and curative healthcare in special circumstances (missions, firing exercises) and health management attributions, my main preoccupation was public health with focus on Frontier Police troops. Among the main objectives we list the following:

- health promotion by sanogenic measures in all units and subunits;
- healthcare by prevention of diseases;
- morbidity control by fighting diseases and their consequences.

We may state that the activity of a military physician belongs to social medicine which is a medical branch and a section of public health, focusing on the health status of the assisted troops, in correlation with influencing risk factors. To sum up, it sets the health diagnosis and etiologic factors.

During that period, I had the possibility to monitor in instruction centres the way recruits adapted to the rigours of army life.

I spent the last two years of daily military life (2000-2001) in the medical practice of the District Police Inspectorate (DPI) having thus the possibility to obtain a global image on the influences of occupational stress factors on the health of the employees of the Ministry of Internal Affairs (MIA). This conclusion was revealed by the studies conducted by epidemiologic methods on the distribution of diseases or of risk factors.

C. The third motivation relates to the fact I was a contemporary of changes produced in the Romanian society after the events in 1989, the transition period and its implications for the troops of the Frontier Police, a true psychology of change. It was and still is a unique historic experience to shift from a centralised economy to democracy and free market, with a radical change required, after 50 years, in material and spiritual culture, the latter having deep scientific, artistic, literary, educational, moral and social conscience roots. While the changes 50 years ago (1948-1958) brought individuals with a mediocre or submediocre instruction level to military structures, at present, most members of military staff have higher education, even if sometimes at a superficial level, with a different perception of stress factors (SF)/stress agents (SA) resulting from these transformations. This is why, after 1990, psychologists were employed in Frontier Police Units, with whom I initiated various studies using psychological tests applied individually or on target groups in order to detect SF/SA influencing the health status of the staff.

I have noticed that psychological factors have an important role in determining certain adaptation disorders, being able to declare that a veritable psychology of health was revealed. This statement can be enforced by the definition given by Iamandescu I.B. to Psychosocial Medicine which „deals with the daily behaviour reported to the individual interaction with the socio-familial-occupational environment, additionally researching psicho-social explanations of health risk factors". The adaptation of individuals to the new society is influenced by multiple factors, the most important being personality structure, temper, mentalities, and last but not least the level of intelligence which, regardless of the educational background of each soldier (medium or higher education) interferes in the different perception of SF/SA. Persons with a lower level of intelligence are incapable of coping with mechanisms aiming at limiting the negative effects of stress agents upon the organism, also having a higher psychological vulnerability. There were situations when young recruits or experienced staff members, due to misadaptation to socio-economic changes and, implicitely, due to changes in the position of each individual, chose to take the extreme solution, i.e. suicide.

D. A fourth motivation, equally important for choosing my PhD topic, was the wish to continue the study on the influences of SF/SA on the general health in order for these to become a preferential field in my professional activity, together with new scientific discoveries increasingly proving that, in medicine, the psychosomatic concept supports the diagnosis and treatment of diseased persons. On the same route, I guided my son, Grigore-Alexandru Popescu, a young surgeon, who supported me in composing and finalising the present work.

In the general practice where I carry out my activity as a family physician, the holistic approach of the patient increases the diagnostic and therapeutic efficiency and at the Kinetotherapy Department of the Drobeta Turnu-Severin University Centre of the University of Craiova where I taught, I found that physical-kinetic techniques are effective methods for stress aleviation in a psycho-somatic context. The physician, the psychologist, the kinetic therapist on one side (the healthcare team) and the patient on the other, collaborate to build a partnership which will contribute to the advance of millenium III psychosomatics.

The Author

2. WHO IS DOCTOR STEFAN ODOBLEJA ?

Stefan Odobleja was born on the 3rd of October 1902 in Izvorul Anestilor, village Valea Hotului, in Mehedinti county, Romania, which today bears the name of Stefan Odobleja.

He went to primary school in his home village, then followed highschool at the „Traian" National College in Drobeta Turnu-Severin.

In 1922 he became a student of the Faculty of Medicine in Bucharest, being awarded a scholarship by the Medical Military Institute. In 1928 he presented his Doctorate thesis entitled „Automoble accidents", elaborated at the Forensic Institute, and he was awarded the title of Doctor in medicine and surgery after presenting his work to a board presided by Prof. Dr. Mina Minovici.

As a military physician, he worked in a series of garrisons in the counties(Braila, Tr.Severin, Lugoj, Dorohoi, Turda, Targoviste, Cernavoda). During that period he began to collaborate with the Military Sanitary Journal, where two of his studies were published, namely „Procedeu practic pentru a împiedica aburirea oglinzilor laringoscopice" (Practical procedure preventing steamy laryngoscopic mirrors), in no.11-12, 1928 and „Aplicaţiile gravitaţiei în terapeutică" (Applications of gravity in therapy), in no. 4, 1929. The second study was a continuation of his research which was the subject of his thesis publicly presented in Bucharest in the summer of 1928, entitled: „Atitudinea corpului şi secreţia sudorală" (Body posture and perspiration). Also, in 1929, he published the study: „Metodă de transonanta toracica" (Thoracic transonance method) where he formulated the so called *law of reversibility* (Buletinul medico-terapeutic – Medical-therapeutic bulletin, the 1st of May 1929).

In 1935, in Lugoj, after editing his paper „La phonoscopie, nouvelle methode d'exploration clinique" (Phonoscopy, a novel method of clinical investigation), which places phonoscopy among the most effective diagnostic methods, he also gives it for publication to Gaston Doin Editors in Paris. Later, he develops some of his ideas in this paper in a study published in Revista sanitara militară (Military Sanitary Journal) no.2 in 1936, under the title „Fonoscopia si semiologia acustica" (Phonoscopy and acoustic semiology). Phonoscopy received the „Medic general doctor Papiu Alexandru" (General physician Dr Papiu Alexandru) prize.

In 1937 he attends the IX-th International Congress of Military Medicine and Pharmacy in Bucharest where he presented the paper: „Demonstration de phonoscopie" (Demonstration of phonoscopy), received with great interest by doctor W.S.Bairbridge, the chief of the American delegation. On this occasion, he distributed to participants an announcement in French of his forthcoming work: „Psychologie consonantiste" (Consonantist psychology).

Hereby we'll offer a short explanatin of the term of phonoscopy introduced by Stefan Odobleja which must be regarded as a precursor of echography also refered to as ultrasonography and diagnostic sonography. He estimated that this term was best suited to acoustic phenomena used at the time in medicine. Stefan Odobleja defines phonoscopy as a novel diagnostic method, an acoustic semiology which must be completed and improved with technological progress, by introducing precision instruments awaiting to be invented, thus intuitively describing our contemporary echographs.

The Academy member systematically studies and experiments the way sound changes its characteristics while crossing the human body, thus enabling the identification of the shape and consistency of various organs and of some processes. These experiments were not conducted using high frequencies (ultrasounds) but with low frequencies produced by „tapping" or „splashing" over various body surfaces. The perception of the modified sound (echo) was done with the ear placed on the opposite side. He explains that betwen 40,000-100,000 vibrations/second, the human ear does not perceieve sounds which are defined as „ultrasonic". Ultrasonic investigation was already used in engineering and for military applications, long time before their application in medicine in the form of echography.

Regarding the continuation of research in the reference field, we must state that ultrasonic energy was first used for medical purposes linked to the relation with patients, by dr. George Ludwig in 1940 at the Naval Medical Research Institute, Bethesda, Maryland. The first purely imagistic application is then achieved by the physician Karl Theodore Dussik (1942-1947) of the Vienna University, as a method he designated as „hyperphonography". Stefan Odobleja already formulated these ideas in 1935.

Between 1937-1938 the scientist is preoccupied to contribute to the improvement of the structure and activity of the Romanian military institutions of which he belonged. In this direction he publishes a series of studies in the journal „Spirit militar modern" (Modern military spirit), such as „Teoria şi practica" (Theory and practice), in no. 1/1938 of the above mentioned journal, approaching the problematic of defining the two notions and their objective interdependence.

In another article published in no. 5-6/1939 of the same journal, under the title „Cantitate şi calitate" (Quantity and quality) he analysed the relation between the two notions and their role in the selection of military staff. He continued his studies on military psychology until the beginning of the war, an example being „Simetria şi dualismul razboiului" (Symmetry and dualism of war).

His main work, „Psychologie consonantiste" (Consonantist psychology) was published in two volumes, in Paris, Libraire Maloins, 1938-1939, totalising 880 pages.

After the war, intending to dedicate himself to research activities, he retires from the army in 1946 and starts elaborating an extensive work, „Logica rezonantei" (Logic of resonance), which he will not finalise.

In 1975, at the third International Congress of Cybernetics, organised in Bucharest, he presented the paper „Cibernetica şi Psihologia consonantistă" (Cybernetics and consonantist psychology), published in the volume of the Congress (Springer Verlag, 1976); in parallel, he was preparing a book on this topic, which was published after his death (Editura Scrisul romanesc, Craiova,1978). As disease prevented him from attending the fourth International Congress of Cybernetics in Amsterdam (21-25 August 1978), he sends a new communication entitled „Diversitate şi unitate in cibernetica" (Diversity and unity in cybernetics), which was presented by eng. Stelian Bajureanu and which brought its author international acknowledgement as precursor of cybernetics. B.H.Rudall of the University of Wales, while presenting the session said: „The paper of dr.Odobleja was very well received...Great interest and appreciation were expressed towards Consonantist psychology".

The Romanian Academy acknowledged the merrits of the scientist Ştefan Odobleja and in 1990 he was awarded the title of post mortem member of the Romanian Academy.

3. THE PSYCHOLOGICAL CONCEPTION OF STEFAN ODOBLEJA

We will present the psychological conception of Stefan Odobleja explained in an introductive study by Eng. Mihai Draganescu, member of the Academy (1929-2010), president of the Romanian Academy (1990-1994) and founder of the department of Science and Technology of Information (1992-1998) and by University Professor dr. Pantelimon Golu. This introductive study was composed for the Romanian translation of „Consonantist psychology", published by Editura Stiintifica si Enciclopedica, Bucuresti, 1982.

„...The herritage left to us by Stefan Odobleja in the field of psychological creation imposes itself not so much by quantity but by its quality and inherent value....

At the end of the second volume of the French edition of „Consonantist psychology", there is an extremely appropriate self-characterisation of the very manner of thinking and writing of Stefan Odobleja on subjects such as psychic, psychological phenomena and other types of connected phenomena – *By its external concision, says the author, by its abbreviations, by the limited number of real examples, by synoptical pictures this book is rather a table of contents, a repertoire or a psychology dictionary, a general plan for a great Treaty of psychology which should include 20-30 volumes.*

The work is indeed a huge dictionary in which all the notions of a modern psychology treaty are included, in a condensed manner, with a tendency to systematic arrangement, with an overall quest for a unification principle: consonance. A preponderantly classificatory vision, with emphasys on dichotomy, reversibility, circular movement. A work conducted with the intention, according to the author, of achieving a maximum of synthesis (unity) and a maximum of analysis (plurality).

Faithful to this principle, Odobleja is very well structuring his psychologic work in a section dedicated to the general theory and another dedicated to practical applications.

Examining the evolution of psychology, Odobleja mentions at the very beginning that there were two directions involved i.e. conception and method. Where conception is concerned, psychology evolves from mysticism and animism to realism and materialism, from transcendent explanation to positive, based on data from biology, mechanics and physics; in terms of method, the evolution starts from subjective introspection towards objective observation and further to the experiment, from descriptions and speculations to systematic organisation and applications, from empirical events to laws and classifications.

A first methodological dimension of Odobleja's work consists of this very historical approach, focused on a critical comparison between the status of psychology with its evolution target. Unrefined and hard to digest, difficult and impure, amorphic and diffuse, scattered and diluted, inconsequent and contradictory, psychology is not a good psychology because, as the author explains, instead of operating with fundamental, general, normal, precise, essential aspects, the accidental, subtle, particular, implicit, pathological, misterious ones are preferred. Such a psychology cannot be regarded as scientific, it is literature, alchemy, magic. For it to matter as a science, psychology must adopt a different strategy to approach its objective i.e based upon merging classifications and synthesis, avoiding vague, imprecise, indefinite aspects, avoiding pedantery, bombastics, verbiage, thinking clearly and vehiculating ideas not just words. It should be a psychology which closely communicates with the other sciences, starting with mechanics and physics, going through the group of biological sciences and reaching morals and logics, simultaneously striving to reach an indepth knowledge of these sciences.

Operating in this spirit which reminds us of the rigour of the cartesian methodology, Odobleja critically apraises various conceptions on the psychic, from empirical and sensorial to mystic and spiritual ones, not excluding, of course, freudists, vitalists, biologists and revealing the error in their representation of the psychic.

Odobleja deals with the diversity of the psychological world in the spirit of unitary and unification principles. Psychic phenomena are not isolated in the Universe, they are not a beginning, an *a priori* given fact, nor are they „queuing" after other categories of phenomena. They are preceded and accompanied by physical, mechanical, chemical, biological, neurological material processes and end up with reactions and response behaviours to external stimuli. This is why, in order to work in a productive manner in the field of psychology, the researcher needs multiple knowledge form the area of sciences dealing with non-psychological phenomena. This explains why, before entering psychological grounds, Odobleja focuses on the physical, the natural, justifiably regarded as a source for the psychic, the „fabric" of which it is tailored, its determinant cause. He also offers a very suggestive picture of correspondences between defining notions of physical and psychological concepts. The psychic, in the author's view, is a division of the physical, one of its varieties, or, in our words, a shape of existence and movement of the objective world, with recurrent effects over the generating term – the physical – which is in its turn changed and reshaped into an effect. Alternatively, according to a definition more pregnantly revealing the concept of Odobleja, the psychcological is a circle of energies, a reversibility, a bidirectional energetic transformant, an association of convex and concave lenses, focusing or dispersing the energy or the physical, in other words fulfilling reception and reaction functions.

According to Odobleja, psychological phenomena are never exclusively interior, direct, immediate. They are triggered by external causes and manifest by physiological, physical and chemical effects. Even such a complex phenomenon as the conscience, with its duplicating and reflexion capacities, has a correspondent in the physical world, in the self-induction process.

From a dynamic point of view, the psychic appears to Odobleja as a complex of processes, states and functions. What would these be? Could these be the three large categories of processes – cognitive, affective, volitional – already inferred by Aristotle and explicitely stated by Christian Wolf and Immanuel Kant? Odobleja rejects this point of view, showing that *the division of the psychic into three slices represents a stereotypical imitation of the teological trinity, an illogical, sterile and stupid trichotomy*. It is not the primitive ramification of the psychic into three components which is logical, real, truthful but the existence of a primary dichotomy, practiced onto the directions of „centripetal psychic" and „centrifugal psychic" – knowledge and will, respectively – followed by a secondary dichotomy consisting of the duplication of the centripetal segment into intelligence and affectivity. The latter, acts as a unity of two opposite poles – pleasure and pain – and knowledge, as a mediating structure in between. This is a truth frequently revealed by modern psychological analysis, namely that affective processes are not reduced to feeling but also inherently contain authentic moments of knowledge. Moreover, Odobleja suggests a complex vision – functionalistic and dialectical – on the relations between the two psychological cathegories and between these and the remaining system in which they are integrated. Such as a dynamo, affectivity is distributed around the internal nature of the organism and it is coupled to it, whereas the cognitive – a dynamo in its turn – is distributed by double contact, between affectivity and the external world, mediating their reciprocal reports. Stefan Odobleja had an exceptional intuition on the psychological truth that introducing knowledge in a relation with affectivity is not acquired according to the continuous series principle but according to the contradiction principle of collaboration from opposite positions, translated into antagonistic pairs: exogenous – endogenous, exteroceptive – interoceptive, objective – subjective, indifferent – appreciative, epicritic – protopathic, etc. While cognition is specialised on the direction of catching the exterior world, affectivity collaborates as a profound, internal dimension of conscience, as a reporting manner, as an attitude.

Focused on thie manner of conceptual organisation, many pages in the work of Odobleja are dedicated to an analytical discussion of cognitive processes with their various subspecies and components, affective and volitional processes, attention, aptitudes, etc. The justified criticism of the anthropomorphic conception which tends to personify psychological processes using tautologic statements such as: „we memorize with our memory", „we think with our thinking", „we perceive with our perception", substituting the person as a true subject by abstract fictions is worth mentioning.

Regardless of the category they belong to, concrete psychological phenomena are subsumed in common existing and functioning principles: *antagonism* and *complementarity, correspondence* and *reversibility.* We find that the consequence with which the author seeks to identify, in various forms of psychological life, the organisation and functioning based upon *binarity, parity, symmetry, bivalence, alternation* is of high methodologic value.

In this direction, the author's considerations regarding the senses qualify in our opinion as prolegomene to a modern study on the psychology of sensitivity. These are regarded as photographic, cinematographic devices of the psychcological „machine" or „factory" – in the author's words – indicating potential differences between the physical exterior and psychological interior, a sort of bridge parapet always separating into two branches (two categories of sensations) the flow of excitations, installations for collecting and releasing physical energy to the nervous centres, bipolar detectors. The author brings numerous examples of grouping sensorial functions according to the model of opposite pairs. They collect, select, transform, amplify or reduce – depending on the circumstance – the energy of external excitations, and sensations which, as the author justifiably observes, constitute a fundament of the entire psychological life, appear as interposed in between excitations and reactions, similarly to the manner in which, according to an appropriate comparison with the physical domain, sensation is the incidence beam which foregoes the reflected beam (reaction). As reaction signifies reversal, sensation is connected to the wider law of reversibility.

Dichotomic division – i.e. the correct one, opposed to the politomic one, which is enumerative and confusing – belongs, according to the author, to all psychological mechanisms, these functioning on the „yes or no", „positive or negative", „it is or it is not" principle. Thus, the parallelisms and antithesis of affectivity: love – hate, pleasure – pain, calm – nervosity, certainty – skepticism, euforia – melancholy, joy – sadness, optimism – pessimism, those of attention: distraction – concentration, and those of thinking: analysis – synthesis, and those of memory: to memorize – to forget, are mentioned.

Due to psycho-physiological, psycho-pathological and psychosociological researches, the function of memory – „cornerstone of conscience" as described by one author – in the overall psychological architecture is well known today. Stefan Odobleja anticipated the conception regarding this role, considering memory as a „psychological film", a multitude of resonating equipments, a sort of a coil which by raveling and unraveling ensures the reversibility of conscience states, the continuous oscillation between internal reduction of experience (during the phase of recording and fixation) and its external amplification or dilatation during the phase of reproduction. The author rejects the idea of a reduction or amplification centre. The two operations – opposed but complimentary – occur by resonance. Here, the idea of self-movement, of functional autonomy is involved, increasingly revealed, presently, by the research on the functional principle of mental action.

I also find that Odobleja's point of view on affectivity is ingenious and advanced, this being concieved as an effect of the refraction of external exciting factors through the concave lens of subjectivity; as a result, the equal and continuous course of external energies is suddenly deviated and fractured on various directions, thus generating the extreme ends of displeasure and pain, and between these – pleasure, as an optimal point, as an average.

Also, one cannot ignore Odobleja's proposed definitions for numerous other psychological concepts, among which we mention perception – an intersensorial consonance, abstraction – a negative attention, generalisation – a mental contagion, imagination – a system of multiple evoking, a chain of consonances, thinking – an internal behaviour, the ideea – a virtual action.

How does Odobleja see the trigger mechanism of psychological phenomena? These are definitely not linked by wires or strings, as thought by associationists, but by resonance. Due to similarities between them, psychological phenomena consonate, mutually and selectively evoke each other, by remote action, as do radiophonic processes. The idea of consonance, antagonism, binarity based functioning was deduced by Odobleja even before the publication of consonantist psychology, in the work dedicated to the phonoscopic method.

The consonance – dissonance pair, both being components of resonance, is involved in all psychological categories, in abstraction and imagination, in perception and generalisation, in expectation and anticipation. Due to this fact, in psychology, as in physics and chemistry – Odobleja explains – nothing is created, nothing is lost, all is transformed, all is reversible.

Stefan Odobleja gradually reaches the structure of a psychology he himself defines, in his later works, as being binary, circular, analogic, similar. Consonance being defined as harmony, the consonantist psychology becomes, according to the author, a *logic of harmony*, or in other words, a science of organisation and self-regulation.

Starting from this rationale, Odobleja draws, in the second part of the paper, a wide applicative picture, obtained by derivation and proliferation from psychological consonance. This picture is not limited to psychological findings but expands towards biology and sociology, political economics and morals, therapeutics and pedagogy.

A generalised psychological vision is thus obtained, a sort of panpsychologism, a reshaping of all sciences using the psychological phenomenon as a template. All special fields are governed by the same general laws – balance, compensation, inverted reaction, alternance, reversibility – with their unification function.

These laws are found in *psychophysiology*, science based upon the reciprocal action betwen organic and psychic (*psychosomatopsychic effect* a.n.), terms which successively function as cause and effect to one another; in *psychopathology* and *psychiatry*, where nervous diseases, various syndromes are binarily explained, by exacerbation to „hyper" or „hypo" and where each consonantist law can find an equivalent in a therapeutic rule; in *interpsychology* (a branch of the field today designated as social psychology), where interpsychological action appears as a reversible physical resonance, and imitation – one of the most expressive interpsychological phenomena – as a complex reversibility, with multiple, staged consonances; in *biology*, where life appears as a vicious circle of reciprocal actions and reactions;

Stefan Odobleja detects and expresses – obviously, in a natural language – the principle of command and control, inherent to all systems, equally living or lifeless, a central principle of modern cybernetics.

It is undoubtedly Odobleja's merit to have discovered these general principles in the field of psychism, by researching humans, trying to decipher the way the senses, the intellect and its inner feelings work, in other words walking on the territory of the most complex types of structures and interactions, taken further as organisation and functioning models for the other categories of phenomena. He radically changed the view on psychological phenomena – going futher than both associationism and behaviourism – he revolutioned psychological science in theory, conception and method, providing it with novel attributes and drawing on this basis, even though not fully aware at that time, the framework for the future field of cybernetics.

Justifiably showing that to measure a psychological phenomenon means to compare it to a constant value, to establish a vicinity and a consonance with a standard, Odobleja examins a series of indicators which, in fact, are non-psychological: *anatomic symptoms, physiological signs, reactions to exciting factors.* His medical background makes him more interested in the physical and physiological mechanisms and less in the manner the psychic fact is constructed, the way it becomes as such.

Thanks to Odobleja, psychology reveals for the first time its virtues as a *pivot* science, a *relay* science, as expressed by cybernetics specialists, an *interdisciplinary node*, as later emphasized by Jean Piaget.

4. THE PSYCHOSOMATIC CONTENT OF STEFAN ODOBLEJA'S WORK

Consonantist psychology was not a book on cybernetics. But, among the fundamehtal laws which, according to Odobleja, rule the physical and psychological components, there is the *law of reversibility*. In modern terms it may be referred to as the law of reverse connection or feedback. This is the great merit of Ştefan Odobleja, i.e. to have discovered the general character of feedback and to have tried to reveal it within the most various processes and phenomena.

The stress in his work initially falls on consonantism for explaining the psychic. In the foreword, Odobleja expresses the intention to systematise psychology around the notion of consonance, together with the objective to reduce the phychic to physics. Gradually, page by page, reversibility (reverse action, reverse connection) gains importance, consonance cannot be achieved without reversibility (in the sense of feedback). The law of reversibility crosses like a red thread the entire work and his whole thinking process. He dedicates five pages to biology (pages 481-485), a chapter we hereby present in order to reveal his holistic, in other words bio-psycho-social (existential), psychosomatic thinking.

„BIOLOGY

Biology is the science of life, the science of the animated or alive kingdom, the science about living creatures.

There is a static biology (morphology, anatomy) and a dynamic one (physiology).

There is a present biology and a historical one (of the past: the natural history of living organisms, evolutive biology).

There is an animal biology (zoology) and a vegetal one (botanics). Many other varieties may be detected:

General or special;   synthetic or analytic;
Phylosophical or practical;   fundamental or accessory;
Speculative or experimental;   casualist or finalist;
Abstract or complex;   materialist or animist;

DEFINITIONS OF BIOLOGICAL CONCEPTS

Life can be defined by many other phenomena: it is defined by mere things.

It has ben defined by *balance;* life is an unstable balance; a balance between interior and exterior; a balance effect of an interior against the external disbalancing causes.

It can especially be defined by *reversibility*; life is a vicious circle of reciprocal actions and reactions. A complex reversibility of physico-chemical phenomena. A *perpetuum mobile* achieved by nature in the detriment of chemical elements and physical energies. A complex of multiple stratified and interwoven cathalitic phenomena. A reversible couple of actions and reactions. A complex phenomenon in which each partial phenomenon is, successively, cause and effect – consequently, a phenomenon producing the ilusion of finalism. A rotation produced by multiple force couples:

assimilation................disassimilation   attraction.................repulsion
reception...................reaction   growth....................division
synthesis...................analysis   pleasure................ pain

Life was defined by *oscillation* (rhythm, periodicity): "life is an undulating evolution of matter"(*V. Conta*).

It has been defined by *transformation* : thus, life would be a transformant for physico-chemical energies".

4.1.Vision of Stefan Odobleja on psycho-physiological mechanisms induced by stress factors/stress agents

The stress factor/stress agent is a conglomerate of heterogeneous stimuli (physical, chemical, biological, psychological) which interact with the human organism at various levels, the cause-effect conversion being made in the area of superior cognitive psychological proceses, with direct or indirect psychological effects, stress being thus triggered as a reaction of the organism with psychosomatic or somatopsychic effects according to the law of reversibility (retroaction, reverse connexion).

Stress factors (SF)/stress agents (SA), generally not alone but in multiple combinations in a situational configuration and by interacting with the subject in question, create a potentially stressful situation which disrupts psychological homeostasis (psychological balance).

The action of SF/SA is harmful when the subject in question responds at emotional level by anxiety and at initially cognitive level by adaptive response, and if new emotional reactions occur psychic stress may be reached.

A.Wells underlines the fact that there is no theory or cognitive model of anxious disturbances, the author choosing the conception of A.T. Beck where the term of cognition refers to an entire series of mechanisms upon which judgement processes rely, and to a certain point to the content of their product known as thoughts.

The basis of the cognitive theory of emotional disturbances is represented by the assumption according to which disfunctions in this area occur and develop due to interpretations people give to etreme events. At the same time, behaviour responses resulting after such interpretations play, in their turn, a role in maintaining emotional disturbances .

Thus, thoughts may become veritable SF/SA, they may induce various types of stress (distress and eustress) a.n.

A.Ellis considers that irrational beliefs represent the source of emotional and behavioural disturbances, these beliefs generating absolute requirements and requests, the latter being the basis for irrational cognition which is the source of emotional disturbances.

B. Arnold thinks that *the intuitive assesemnt of a situation initiates a tendency to action which is experienced as an emotion and is expressed by various organic changes.*

R.S. Lazarus et al were the first to show the importance of cognitive processes in the genesis of SP and described a general frame for the interaction between SA and the individual, capable to suggest that both the evaluation and reevaluation processes of the harmfulness of SF/SA, as well as the adaptive alternatives, have a major affective resonance.

Describing the dynamics of emotion, B. Arnold identifies a succession of operations which might not reach the equivalent amplitute of a SP. These operations are usually run at the level of the subject's conscience and have the following sequence: perception of SF/SA, memory of similar experiences, reassessment of the situation, actual action.

The occurence of a SF/SA triggers a brain activation which causes a state of emotional tension, generating anxiety when the action persists without an adequate response, the *stress threshold* being thus reached. In this moment, the subject perceives the danger and is either task-oriented, seeking to solve the situation, or self-oriented, tending to maintain the initial psychological balance. Thus, in a first stage, an adaptative mobilization is recorded by improved performance, and during the second stage deteriorated responses occur due to decreased performances and the rigidity of adaptative acts characterised by the incapacity to capitalise previous experience, by the occurence of instability, suspicion, hostility. All these lead to a state of internal conflict described as *exhaustion threshold* characterised by fatigue, ineffectiveness, hopelessness, sense of guilt, in one word *depression* .

SF/SA have a global action before the response is elaborated (primary character) and another one during and after the response is triggered (secondary character), both actions being based upon the principle of reverse connexion, described as influencing the system's state of reception to a new action or to the persistent action of a SA .

4.2. Law of reversibility (retroaction, reverse connexion) governs the entire work of St. Odobleja „Consonantist Psychology" and his entire thinking, he being the one to detect the general character of feedback and to try to highlight it in the most variate processes and phenomena. In this work composed before 1938, probably between 1934-1937, we surprisingly identify in the chapters on *static psychic* (senses, reaction organs, memory), *dynamic psychic*, *fundamental phenomena* (excitations, sensations, reactions), *affective phenomena*, resemblances with the general adaptation syndrome (GAS) described by H. Selye, promoting original ideas, definitions, concepts, laws.

Thus, according to the conception of St.Odobleja, the *excitations* we may assimilate to SF/SA produce, through our senses, sensations which in their turn produce various reactions from the human organism such as adaptative and non-adaptative ones (fig.1).

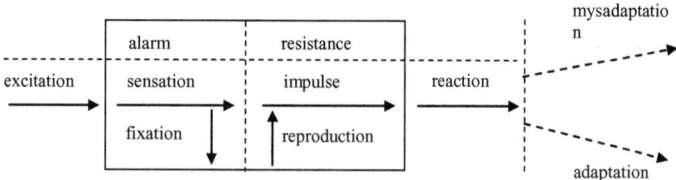

Fig. 1. Possible reactions to SF/SA

Diagram adapted after: Dr. St. Odobleja, *Psychologie Consonantiste,* first volume, Libraire Maloine, Paris, 1938, p. 137.

Fig.1 - „sensation is the internal part of excitation, similarly to the impuls being the interior (psychic) portion of reaction. Fixation is a standstill while reproduction is a restart of the interrupted movement."

In this diagram, fixation (standstill) would be interpreted as an adaptation of the organism to the action of SF/SA, and reproduction and impulse would be the continuation of the action of SF/SA upon the organism, with psychic implications.

Together with physico-chemical excitants, St. Odobleja also considers psychic excitants (images, thoughts, defining senses as „ ... organs of sensations; providers of the psychic, of memory, the entrance gate to the psychic. Contact point for the physic and psychicological components".

For St. Odobleja the universe is a circle (fig. 2), and its two halves are represented by the physic and psychlogical components; „the physic is the source of the psychic and its last expression, its cause and often, its effect, the material of which the psychic is constructed" . Quantitatively, he considers that physique is the largest portion of the universe, it is the „exterior, the periphery, the large sphere; the psychic is the interior, the centre, the smallest portion but the most important in each being's universe".

Fig. 2. The universe seen by St.Odobleja;

From dichotomous divisions which are in fact the basis for the author's conception, we may observe that the origin of excitants and reactions lies within the physique:

Transformable physique, pre-psychic, excitants;
Transformed physique, post-psychic, reactions and acts

SA/SF are originally either physico-chemical or they are psychlogical stimuli finally acting at psychic level where the impulse as a psychic phenomenon is produced which will trigger reactions belonging to the physiological area. At psychic level, affective phenomena St. Odobleja describes as concepts, intervene as an effect of external excitants' refraction through the concave lens of the organism's subjectivity, process during which the even and continuous course of external energies is suddenly deviated in different directions, thus generating the external poles of inconvenience and pain with pleasure situated betwen them (fig.3).

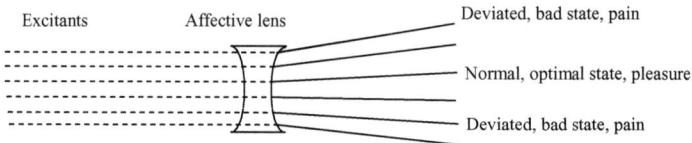

Fig. 3. Affective lens; Source: op. cit., p.158

We may state without being mistaken that in his work, St. Odobleja originally describes the psycho-physiological mechanisms triggered in the organism by various external or internal stimuli, as well as the importance of the psychic in the adaptation or inadaptation processes of the organism to these stimuli.

Presently, the multiple reactions of the psycho-somatic system triggered by internal or external stimuli with different sources have been elucidated. The psycho-physiological unity of the human organism obliges us to regard stress rather as somatopsychic or psychosomatic, and we must avoid refering to somatic and/or psychic stress.

The information comming from inside or outside the organism influences the synthesis of pituitary neurohormones which will in their turn influence the secretion of peripheral hormones which will then act upon various tissues. Upon the assessment of the stressful character all the elements of the nervous system intervene (v. fig.4).

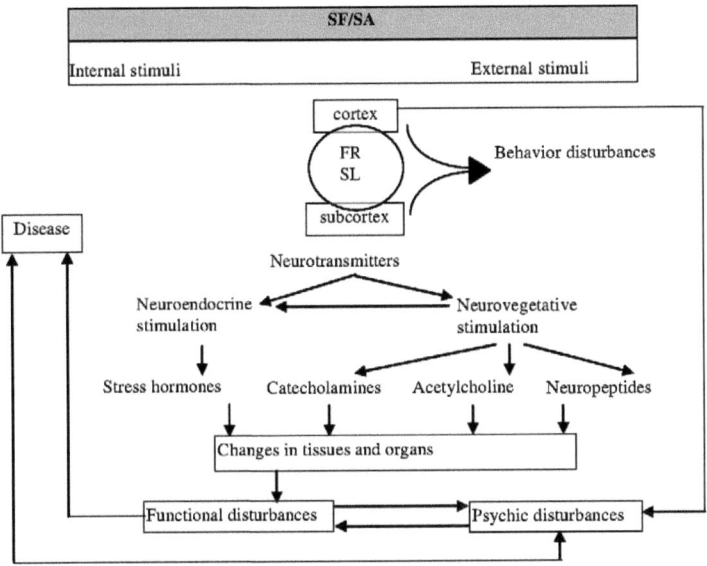

Fig. 4. Neurohormonal reactions and PSD (psycho-somatic disorders) produced by SF/SA

Surce adapted after: I.B. Iamandescu (1999): *Elemente de psihosomatica*, Ed. INFOmedica, Bucuresti, p.44

Mac Lean and V. Reichlin, classify neurovegetative fibers into three large categories: *sympathetic* (adrenergic), *parasympathetic* and *non- adrenergic, non – cholinergic*. The latter, even though vehiculated by sympathetic or parasympathetic nerves, have different neurotransmitters. The stimulation of sympathetic and parasympathetic nerves is not entirely blocked by antiadrenergic and anticholinergic drugs, suggesting the existance of certain nervous fibers with other neurotransmitters .

Accoding to St.Odobleja, the vegetative nervous system (VNS) is the coordinating, normalising, compensatory organ reacting against disbalances. When discussing the criticism of the vago-sympathetic theory, he shows that it evolved from the dogmatic systematisation of Eppinger and Guillaume and the amphotropism of Danielopolu and explains that the theory „...neglects the existence of peripheral organs, their individuality, their direct and non-mediated reciprocal actions, direct (peripheroperipheral) nervous correlations between various organs are neglected: nothing is mentioned on direct relations and interactions from one organ to another. Only top to bottom actions are admitted as well as those exerted by means of the vago-sympathetic nervous system."; „in reality, there is no inhibitory system opposing an excitant system: each nervous fillet is successively inhibitor and exciter. From this stand point, each nervous fillet is an indifferent conductor, also each nervous cell (or ganglion) react either by excitation or by depression – case by case, depending on the excitant, on its dose, on the physiological state, etc.".

Of those above presented, the idea that St. Odobleja had an integrative vision on the activity of the two vegetative systems, the sympathetic and parasympathetic, emerges.

In his conception, the brain is an energy resonator, and sensorial organs are collectors, selectors, transformers, amplifiers and reductors, resonators-receptors, resonators-amplifiers, captating excitations (SF/SA) and transforming them into psychic energy which would be of unknown origin, probably transmitted by some endocrine secretions (neurotransmitters, neuromodulators) producing the condensation of peripheral excitations with central decondensation or detension or vice-versa, process which according to the consonance/disonance theory would lead to disbalances which endanger the psychic, endocrine and, finally, the general homeostasis.

Regardless of the number and variety of stressors, the human organism only has one type of physiological defense mechanism and this mainly depends on the integrity of the corticosuprarenal gland whose hyperactivity is responsible of adaptation disturbances, the human organism being the victim of its own biological defense mechanisms.

5. CONSONANTIST PSYCHOSOMATICS

The title *Consonantist Psychosomatics* is intended to highlight the contribution of Doctor Stefan Odobleja to the psychosomatics concept which was already underlined in antiquity by Hippocrates.

In his work entitled „Consonantist Psychology", with the aid of nine universal laws, based upon the resonance phenomenon and energetic psychological processes, the creator of generalized cybernetics designs a new model for a psychosomatic approach rendering a cosmic side to the bio-psycho-social model.

The title is a syntagm composed of two words: psychosomatics and consonantism, these being connected by subordinance as well as by correlation of meaning. We may state they may be considered a stable syntactic unit.

From this point of view, the place and role of the great scientist Şt.Odobleja in the history of psychosomatics may be established.

Psychosomatics is a medical approach connecting psychological and somatic aspects.

Consonance is defined by Odobleja as a „physical phenomenon characterized by similitude, selectivity and movement (or vibration) ... a reversible excitation. A reversibility, a reciprocity, a mutual classification. The identity principle (similitude) and the excluded third party (selectivity) reduced to the physical phenomenon of resonance, a complex phenomenon, caused by sense and frequency similitude with effects of: selectivity, excitation, fusion. The totality of selectivity, amplification, dynamogenics and fusion phenomena produced by superposition of two movements, vibrations similar or related by their direction and frequency".

Among the multiple classes of consonance, Odobleja denominates a physical-psychological and a psychological-physical consonance, i.e. psycho-somatic and somatic-psychological

Brief history: The psychosomatic unity was underlined as early as Antiquity by Hippocrates, being a concept regarding the human being as a whole, somatic and psychological components being closely interdependent and disease being considered as an individual reaction to the environment.

Anaxagora (504-428 B.C.) was among the first to speak about psychological-somatic dualism (mind-body relation) which was developed by the great Greek antique philosophers Plato and Aristotle: „the soul gives shape to the body and becomes its vital principle"...

The psycho-somatic unity is also found in the middle Ages in philosophers (XVII-th – XVIII-th centuries) such as Descartes, Hobbes, Berkley, and Leibnitz.

The first to talk about psychosomatics in modern times is Heinroth (1818) who was also the one to introduce the term of „somatopsyche" in 1828.

In 1890, Sommer introduces the term of psychogenesis which will be adopted and supported by the great creators of psychogenesis theories (P.Janet Freud).

In 1899, Pavlov describes the influence of emotions on physiological processes, conditional reflexes.

In 1912, Adler argued in favor of holism, analyzing the individual rather from the perspective of the entire psychological existence.

In 1922, Deutsch presents the organ neurosis.

Psychosomatics was introduced as a medical term in the period between 1936-1938 when the first psychosomatics societies emerge and the first specific journals are published.

It is worth mentioning that during the same period, i.e. in the year 1938, the first volume of the French version of consonantist psychology was published in Lugoj and distributed through „Libraire Maloine" in Paris and in 1939 the second volume was published, both volumes being distributed to great universities in the world.

We further mention the personalities who contributed to the field of modern psychosomatics: 1943 - Helen Fl. Dunbar with specific personality profiles for each psychosomatic disorder; 1946 - Hans Selye with the general adaptation syndrome; 1950 - Alexander with conflict specificity; 1957 - Hinkle, Wolff with the determinant role of environmental factors and others such as von Uexkull, Schafer, Sifneos, Batson, Basedovsky, etc.

The encyclopedic dictionary describes Stefan Odobleja as „...author of the first variant of the generalized cybernetic concept, trying to explain natural phenomena, and especially those of biology and psychology, by inverse connection (law of reversibility)...notices and highlights the phenomenon of adaptation of living organisms to environmental conditions", aspect introduced by Hans Selye in 1946. These aspects may be considered a proof of his connection to psychosomatics.

As a synthesis, we may state that this concept has passed through several distinct stages in time.

The first Hippocratic stage describes the relation between mind (psyche) and body (soma).

The second stage begins in 1890 with Sommer, who introduces the term of psychogenesis in this relation.

The third stage starts with the modern era when the existential ecological environment is integrated into the psyche-soma unit, i.e. the bio-psycho-social model of Engel - 1974. But in order to establish the starting point of this stage we must go back to the year 1939 when Odobleja, with his work „Consonantist Psychology" and by the law of reversibility (feedback) brings an essential contribution to the psycho-somatic unit by establishing a mutual psycho-somatic relationship. By multi- and interdisciplinary arguments, he expands the psycho-somatic approach of the human being in the universe. He, thus, creates a novel model, connecting the bio-psycho-social model to the universe by the nine universal laws (equivalence, equilibrium, compensation, reaction, oscillation, inertia, transformation, consonance, reversibility) which he harmonized into a consonance/resonance based upon the law of reversibility and psychological energetic processes for all human life phenomena. He performs an in-depth analysis of the connection between mind, body and universe, rendering a cosmic side to the model. The psychosomatic approach from a consonantist psychology perspective is demonstrated by Stefan Odobleja by defining psychological and physical components.

Thus, the physical component is described as the nature, the outside world. „ The physical component is the source of psyche and its ultimate expression, cause and, often effect, the fabric of which psyche is made. It is one of the first opposing categories of psyche. From a logical point of view, the physical component is one of the halves of the universe, the other one being the psyche; quantitatively, it is by far the largest part of the universe.

The physical component is the exterior, the periphery, the larger sphere; psyche is the inside, the centre, the smaller but the most important portion of each being's universe".

By describing the physical divisions the author analyzes the physical as the exterior, i.e. the universe but also the human being, with mutual influences between them.

„ Psychologically, the physical component is classified as:

- transformable, pre-psyche, excitants;
- transformed, post-psyche, reactions and acts...

Biologically, the classification includes:
- the inert nature: the lifeless objects, the physical component per se;
- the living nature: the beings, the biological".

Further, Odobleja states that the physical component is studied by natural sciences:
- for lifeless nature (cosmological sciences) he describes static sciences (chemistry, geography, mineralogy, astronomy, etc.) and dynamic sciences (physics, mechanics, sky mechanics, etc. – quantum mechanics might be added here)
- for living nature (biological sciences) he similarly describes static sciences (anatomy, histology) and dynamic sciences (physiology, evolution)".

Also, the author considers that any psychology must include an introductory study on physics for the following reasons:

1.,, The physical always precedes and determines the psyche, thus constituting its cause:
- static causes: - anatomic-histological substrate (the brain)
                 - chemical composition of the substrate
- dynamic causes: - physical excitants
                  - physiological excitants

2. The physical follows the psyche: it represents its effect; we are thus obliged to study it:
- as a material, static effect: - anatomical, structural
                                - chemical, constitutional
- as an energetic, dynamic effect: - psychically determined physical phenomena
                                   - determined physiological phenomena

3. The physical resembles the psyche which confounds with it in several aspects: statically, the psyche may be attributed to a biological structure and to a chemical constitution; dynamically, psychological phenomena are reducible, as a whole, to physical phenomena.

Odobleja describes the psyche as being the soul, the spirit, the inner universe, as a biological function located in the brain. ,, As any other function, the psyche serves life;

34

it is correlated to each of the other functions of the organism (psycho-physiological correlations). It is strictly dependent to a system of organs. Psychological phenomena are very strictly dependent on circulation and on the physiological status of the organism at a certain moment. Psychological activity is influenced by physical, chemical and biotic agents". To conclude, Odobleja is the first physician to state that the true elements of psychological phenomena are invisible – as are the elements or material substrate of physical energies – and analogical, if not identical with the latter. The psychological process is no longer such a rudimentary phenomenon as the presumed mechanical vicinity and removal of neuronal fibers – but an extremely fine, energetic process". This invisible, energetic, vibration element, intuitively described by Odobleja, is described as „string" by some contemporary physicists.

In subchapter on psycho-physiology, the author defines it as a study of „reciprocal repercussions (interactions) between centre and the periphery, between physical and physiological, between moral and body, between brain and the other viscera, between general and local, between the whole and its parts; the science of psycho-physical reactions. Each organ has relations with all the other organs, including the brain. The brain is, undoubtedly, a privileged organ but it does not hold the monopole on inter-organic communications".

He also describes the influences of psyche upon the psychological component, which are: „ reversible (functional – in fact, psychosomatic disorders) or irreversible (organic – in fact, psychosomatic diseases); normal (physiological) or abnormal (pathological); and the influences of the physiological components upon the psyche (somatic-psychic action) which also classifies them into reversible and irreversible; normal or pathological, durable or transient".

Odobleja also mentions that between the physical component and the psyche, between body and soul, there is a mutual influence: each is in its turn cause and effect and he introduces the more accurate notion of reciprocal influence between each body part and each part of the psyche.

We may state that the work of the scientist has opened a new perspective for the development of the psychosomatic concept.

In the bibliography studied by Odobleja for his work, which includes 700 papers, we find names of authors cited during the history of psychosomatics such as: Janet P

(1891), Adler (1924), Pieron (1927), Pavlov (1932), Marinescu (1910), Descartes, Freud.

After the book „Consonantist Psychology" was published in 1939, in his manuscripts, titles of works on the psychosomatic concept and the atomic universe were found, such as: „Psychosomatic medicine – insights in medical enigmas", Bonneton Andre, Paris, Libraire Maloine, (1964) and „Man and the atomic universe", Coudures E, 1951. This demonstrates that he continued to be concerned and studied the way the physical and psychological components influence one another. Odobleja considers that „the true elements of psychological phenomena are invisible – as are the elements or the material substrate of physical energies – and analogical, if not identical with the latter".

Nowadays, a lot is said on the psychology of order – quantum psychology (POQP), which is an interdisciplinary synergistic science, built on information from philosophy, psychology, informatics, medicine, physics, biology, cybernetics. POQP seeks the systemic-holistic knowledge of the human psyche universe by means of original measurement instruments and methodologies, based on the generalized quantum theory, in order to optimize human condition from the perspective of the existential purpose and of psycho-somatic and psychological health. Other fields are also mentioned such as quantum medicine, quantum neuroscience and, if all these were to be based on quantum psychology, we might state another syntagm i.e. **quantum psychosomatics**.

Among the few who mention Stefan Odobleja and his contribution in this area of quantum enigmas, Prof. Ion Manzat, president of the Romanian Association of Transpersonal Psychology, defines psychological resonance (intuitively described by Stefan Odobleja) as a transpersonal energy vibration explained by expanded psycho-synergy.

The main merit of Odobleja is that of intuitively describing the fundamental structure connecting humans to nature (that invisible, energetic, vibration element which physicists describe as „**string**". His work radiates a cosmic thinking on life dynamics and is a true resource for ideas in the third millennium.

The value of his work on the psychosomatic concept passed unnoticed during his time. Hopefully, from now on, by our actions, we shall restore the well deserved place in the history of national and international medicine and continue to study his published work and manuscripts kept by the State Archives.

6. CONSONANTIST PSYCHOLOGY – A PSYCHO-SOMATO-PSYCHOLOGICAL APPROACH

Between 25-28 June 2014 Sibiu hosted the annual meeting of the European Association of Psychosomatic Medicine „Care and Cure – an integrated approach to psychosomatic medicine", accredited by the European Accreditation Council for Continuous Medical Education.

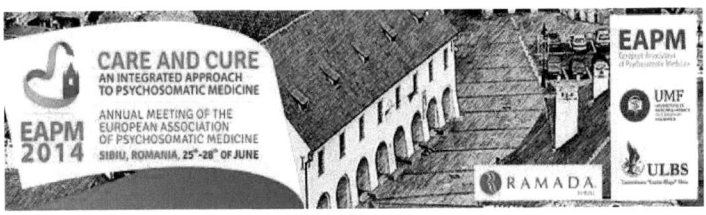

EAPM-2014 (fig.5) was a great success:
- 270 participants from 39 countries on 5 continents;
- Over 210 presented paper abstracts from 35 countries;
- 19 symposia included in the program;
- 6 plenary sessions;
- over 80 poster presentations in 2 plenary sessions.

During the first plenary session I presented a poster (fig. 6- Univ. Prof. DHC Liviu Sofonea, President of the Romanian Committee for History of Philosophy, Science and Technology of the Romanian Academy, left and Dr. Nicolae Popescu, right) in which I highlighted the medical applications of the works of St. Odobleja and the contribution to the concept of psychosomatics. For a synthetic approach of the ideas, thesis and concepts demonstrating that „Consonantist Psychology" is in fact a psycho-somato-psychological approach usable in medicine, we introduced the syntagm of „Consonantist Psychosomatics".

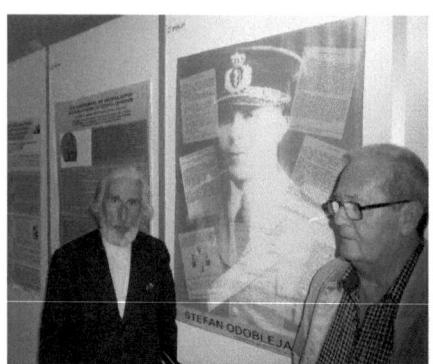

Fig.6

Analytical study investigating the relations and inter-relations between psychosomatics and consonantist psychosomatics. Academy Member Stefan Odobleja, army physician, internationally acknowledged as the parent of generalized cybernetics and creator of psycho-cybernetics, deserves a special place in the history of both cybernetics and psychosomatics. The work *Psychologie consonantiste* (880 pp), published in French in Lugoj, in two volumes, during 1938-1939, was distributed by Librairie Maloine in Paris. In 1978 at the International Congress of Cybernetics and Systems in Amsterdam, 30 years of cybernetics were celebrated and the „Norbert Wiener" medal was inaugurated. Upon this occasion Stefan Odobleja's world priority on the idea of generalized cybernetics was acknowledged, 10 years prior to N.Wiener, whose cybernetics is in fact a technical application of general cybernetics.

„THE PSYCHOLOGICAL (the soul, the spirit, the interior universe)...

THE PSYCHOLOGICAL IS A BIOLOGICAL FUNCTION LOCATED IN THE BRAIN.

...any physiology is ultimately reduced to physical and chemical. Do the psychological belong to the physical or chemical? *And, if the former is true,* does it belong to the *mechanical* – as taught by all psychology manuals – or is it *energetic,* of a more subtle and superior nature than a vulgar act of fibre contact?...

The true elements of psychological phenomena are invisible – as are the elements or material substrate of physical energies – and analogue, if not identical, with the latter. The psychological process is no longer such a vulgar phenomenon as the supposed mechanical approaching and coming apart movements of neuronal fibres – but an extremely fine tuned process, an energetic process.

38

Psychology really is the physiology of nervous centres, but it is only the most refined, intimate, subtle part of this physiology: the rest is neurology. *Psychology is a physiology without anatomy,* as its true anatomy, the veritable psychological anatomy i.e. energetic microscopy has not yet been inaugurated. Until new developments, we can only mentally represent it, by imitating chemists and physicists who do the same for valences, atoms, quanta, ions and their electrons. Maybe man will never be able to see and directly observe by his senses – including devices which enhance them – the true material-anatomic substrate of his psychology." (Odobleja St. -premier volume 1938-, Psychologie consonantiste, premier et deuxieme volume, Libraire Maloine, Paris, p.p. 51-64).

„DEFINITIONS

The physical body is the source of the psychological and its ultimate expression, cause and, often, effect, the material the psychological is made of. It is one of the first categories, opposed to the psychological. From a logical perspective, the physical body is one of the two halves of the Universe, the other being the psychological: quantitatively it is by far the largest part of the Universe…

DIVISIONS OF THE PHYSICAL

Psychologically, we must make the distinction between:
-   the transformable physical, the pre-psychological, the excitants;
-   the transformed physical, the post-psychological, the reactions and acts.

From the perspective of change:
-   the static physical: the matter, the substance, the chemical, the structure, the anatomy;
-   the dynamic physical: the energy, the force, the actual physical, the phenomena, the function, the physiological.

From a biological perspective:
-   the inanimate nature: lifeless bodies, the actual physical;
-   the living nature: the beings, the biological.

The study of the physical belongs to natural sciences:

- for inanimate nature: cosmological sciences

  static: chemistry, geography, mineralogy, astronomy, etc.

  dynamic: physics, mechanics, sky mechanics, etc.
- for living nature: biological sciences:

  static: anatomy, histology

  dynamic: physiology, evolution."

(Odobleja St. -premier volume 1938-, Psychologie consonantiste, premier et deuxieme volume, Libraire Maloine, Paris, p.p.47-48).

„PSYCHOLOGY (general notions)

DEFINITION

Psychology is the science of the soul, of the conscience, of conscience phenomena; the science of non-mediated facts, of interior experience, of psychological facts or phenomena, a science derived from introspection (genetic, empirical, sensualist, and subjective definition). It is the science of sciences, the key and fundament of all the other sciences and of philosophy (a noologic definition by its effects). It is the physiology of the brain; central and fine tuned physiology of the relation apparatus (objective, biological, anatomic-physiological definition). It is the science of *reciprocal actions* exerted by stimulation, adaptation, or adjustment and response between an organism and the environment (H. Spencer and behavior psychology). It is *brain physics: the science of internally perceived physical phenomena (propagations, balances and unbalances, consonances and dissonances, actions and reactions, loads and unloads, etc.* physical concept, supported in the present paper)...

Psychophysics

According to the old, limited and restricted concept, psychophysics is the science of reports between sensations and their exciting triggers. More widely defined, psychophysics is a synthesis between psychological and physical, the definition of the psychological with the aid of the physical, the physicist concept on the physical, the knowledge of the psychological unknown through the known physical, the unification of psychological sciences and physical or natural sciences, the equivalence of physical and psychological sciences with the consequent application of methods and devices from physics in the field of the psychological, and the use of experimental method. Our psychology is ultimately psychophysics in a wider sense: it is psychological physics".(Odobleja St. -premier volume 1938-, Psychologie consonantiste, premier et deuxieme volume, Libraire Maloine, Paris, p.p.39, 46).

„ PSYCHO - NEUROLOGY

Neurology is sometimes understood as a subordinate of psychology; it would be the study of anatomy, physiology, pathology, etc. of the nervous system (including the study of the brain and of psychology). It may also be understood as a subordinate of physiology: in this case neurology would be the study of transmissions, the science of connections between soul and body, between centre and periphery, between psychological and physical...

The influences of the psychological upon the physiological (psycho-somatic effects) are:

Reversible (functional) – psychosomatic dysfunctions n.a. – or irreversible (organic) – psychosomatic diseases n.a. - Normal (physiological) or abnormal (pathological). Durable (evolutive, permanent, anatomic, organized: physiognomy, voice, conformation, gaining or losing weight etc.) or short lasting (transitory, functional: mimic, gestures, expressions, attitudes, manners, hand writing etc.). Intense or weak; Mediated or immediate; Direct or indirect; Local or diffuse; Excitant (dynamogenic, stimulating, sthenic) or depressing (calming, asthenic, inhibitory); Motor or secretor; Induced by sensations or by representations – cognitive or affective.

The influences of the physiological upon the psychological (somatic-psychological effects n.a.) are reversible or irreversible; normal or pathologic; durable or transient; strong or weak; local or diffuse, excitant or depressing etc. There are effects on receptivity and effects on reaction; effects on the intelligence and effects on affectivity.

...Does the physical determine the psychological or is it the other way around? In reality, between centre and periphery there is reciprocity of action, there are reciprocal interactions, balancing oscillations in alternative current. Between physical and psychological, between body and soul there is a reciprocal influence: each is, in its turn, cause and effect.

Is this influence vague or precise? We must replace the vague notion of reciprocal influence of physical and moral, by the more precise notion of reciprocal influences between each body part and each psychological component." (Odobleja Șt. -premier volume 1938-, Psychologie consonantiste, premier et deuxieme volume, Libraire Maloine, Paris, p.p. 407, 426,427).

41

„ PSYCHO-SOMATIC INTERACTIONS

Definition: Psycho-physiology is the study of reciprocal repercussions (interactions) between centre and periphery, between physical and psychological, between moral and body, between brain and the other viscera, between general and local, between the whole and its components. It is the study of psycho-somatic reflexes; the science of psycho-somatic interactions (fig7).

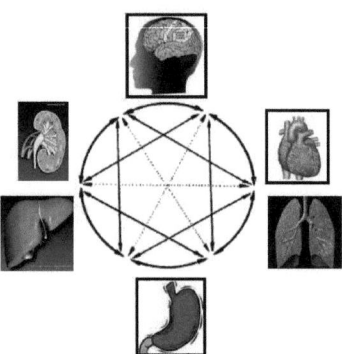

Fig.7: Psycho-somatic interactions. Source: adapted after Şt.Odobleja (1939): Psychologie consonantiste, deuxième volume, Libraire Maloine, 27, rue de L'école-de-médecine 27, Paris ,1939

There are inter-organic actions achieved by nervous centres (brain, heart, lungs, stomach, intestines, liver, kidneys, and sexual organs). There are also direct inter-organic actions. Each organ has relations with every other organ, including the brain. The brain is, undoubtedly, a privileged organ, but it does not hold exclusivity on inter-organic communication". (Odobleja Şt.-premier volume 1938-, Psychologie consonantiste, premier et deuxieme volume, Libraire Maloine, Paris, p.535).

Throughout its vast content, the work „Psihologia consonantistă" (Consonantist psychology), uses nine universal laws i.e. those of equivalence, equilibrium, compensation, reaction, oscillation, reversibility, inertia, consonance, transformation, all based upon the resonance phenomenon. He was the first attempting to apply the feedback law (law of reversibility) in nature and society, in as many scientific fields as possible: philosophy, biology, psychology, sociology, political economics, mathematics and even medicine (psycho-neurology, psychophysiology, psychopathology, interpsychology), enabling an easier understanding of the interrelations between biological, psychological and social factors, of the psycho-somatic connections in the practice of psychosomatic medicine.

The syntagm of consonantist psychosomatics facilitates a better understanding of the psychosomatic circuit, psycho-physiologically and clinically expressed in the work of Stefan Odobleja.

7. HISTORY PSYCHOSOMATICS

> - Unity psyche-soma-underlined antiquity (Hipocrates)
> - Century philosophers-XVII-Descartes, Spinoza, Leibniz mind body relationship (dualism)
> - Johann Christian Heinroth(1773,1843)-inventor of the term „psychosomatic"
> - 1843, Cabanis-relations betwween the physical and moral
> - 1885, Freud – courts personality, levels of awareness of mental processes, stages of instinctual development,transfer psychoanalysis
> - 1892, Fere – pathology emotions
> - 1899, Pavlov – concussion influence on psysiological processes, conditioned reflexes
> - 1912, Adler – locus minoris resistentiae
> - 1922, Deutsch – organ neuroses
> - 1938 ,1939 , Odobleja – Psychology Consonantiste
> - 1943, Fl. Dumbar – specific personality profiles for each BPS
> - 1946, Selye – General Adaptation Syndrome
> - 1950, Alexander – specific conflict
> - 1955, EY- organ neurosis and psychosomatic medicine
> - 1956, Silva – psychosomatic medicine
> - 1956, Kaplan – psychosomatic medicine,the importance of psychological factors in medicine
> - 1957, Hinkle, Wolff – environmental factors = role
> - 1959, Grinker and Robbinns – psychosomatic clinic
> - 1963, Von Uexkull – differentiation of conversion disorder
> - 1963, Marty, M' Uzan – thinking operative
> - 1964, Tzank –general practice/family medicine (MG/MF) is a true psychosomatic medicine
> - 1965, Klotz – Psychosomatic Medicine is the most elaborate MG/MF
> - 1966, Schafer – sociopsihosomatica

> 1969, Scheneider – Medical Psychology
> 1973, Sifneos, Nemiah – alexithymia
> 1974, Bateson – general systems theory
> 1979, Von Eieff – neurogenic hypertension
> 1981, 1985, Locke, Besedovsky – SP involvement in the functioning of the immune system (psychoneuroimmunology)

Adapted from: Dr. Diaconescu L., quoted by I.B.Iamandescu (1999): Elements of General and Applied psychosomatic, Ed Infomedia,Bucharest, PP2-3.

8. REFERENCES

1. ARNOLD B.MAGDA (1970): *Feeling and emotions*, Academic Press, New-York.

2. ARNOLD B. MAGDA (1960): *Emotion and personality*, University Press, New - York, Chicago.

3. BECK A.T. (1976): *cognitive Therapy and the Emotional Disordes*, International University Press, New-York.

4. DUMITRASCU D.L., SOELLNER W. (2014), proceedings of EAPM 2014, *Care and cure – an integrated approach to psychosomatic medicine*, Annual meeting of the European Association of Psychosomatic Medicine, MEDIMOND - monduzzi editore International Proceedings Division.

5. ELLIS A.GRIEGER R. (1977): *Handbook of Rationale therapy*, Springer Corp, New-York.

6. HOLDEVICI I. (2002): Psihoterapia anxietatii - Abordari cognitiv comportamentale, Ed.Dual Tech,Bucuresti.

7. IAMANDESCU I.B. (1993) : *Stresul psihic și bolile interne*, Ed.All, Bucureşti.

8. IAMNADESCU I.B. (1999): Elemente de psihosomatica generala si aplicata,Ed.INFOmedica,Bucuresti.

9. KUTTNER F.,ROSENBLUM B. (2011); Enigma cuantica,fizica intalneste constiinta,Ed.Prestige,Bucuresti.

10. LAZARUS R.S. (1969*): Psychological stress and coping process*, New-York, McGroww-Hill.

11. ODOBLEJA ST. .(1938): *Psychologie Consonantiste*, premiere volume, Librairie Maloine, 27, rue de L'ecole de medecine, Paris.

12. ODOBLEJA ST. (1982): *Psihologia Consonantistă*, Ed.Ştiinţifică şi Pedagogică, Bucureşti.

13. ODOBLEJA ST. (1935): La phonoscopie, novelle méthode d'exploration clinique, G. Doin & Cie, Editeurs, Paris.
14. POPESCU N. *Doctor Şt.Odobleja*, Medicina in Evoluţie, Nr.1, Ed.Sigma Plus, Deva.
15. POPESCU N.,CENEA M. (2006), Factorii de stres si patologia psihosomatica,teorii si cercetari la nivel organizational, Ed.Universitaria,Craiova.
16. POPESCU N., POPESCU G.A. (2013), *Vision of Stefan Odobleja on psycho-physiological mechanisms induced by stress factors/stress agents,* Medicine in evolution, nr. 4, 2013, Timisoara.
17. WELLS A. (1999): *Cognitive Therapy of Anxiety Disorders,* John and Sones Chichester, New-York, Weinheim, Brisbane, Singapore, Toronto, 3rd Edition.

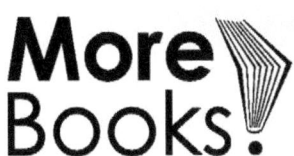
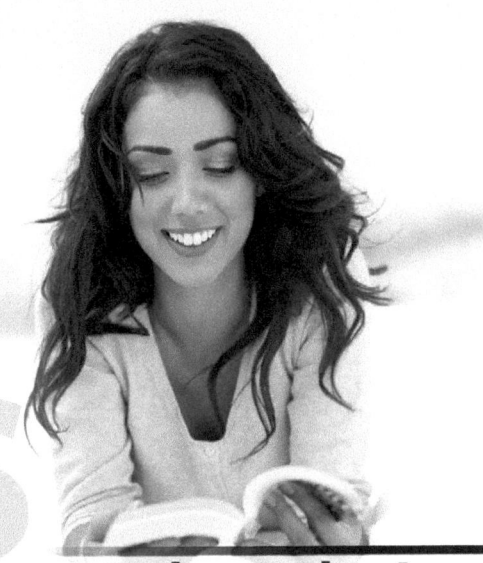
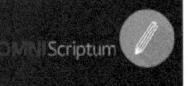

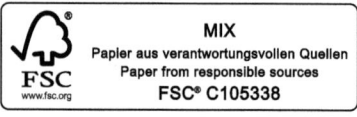